Enjoy The Sound Of

Pump it up

RADIO

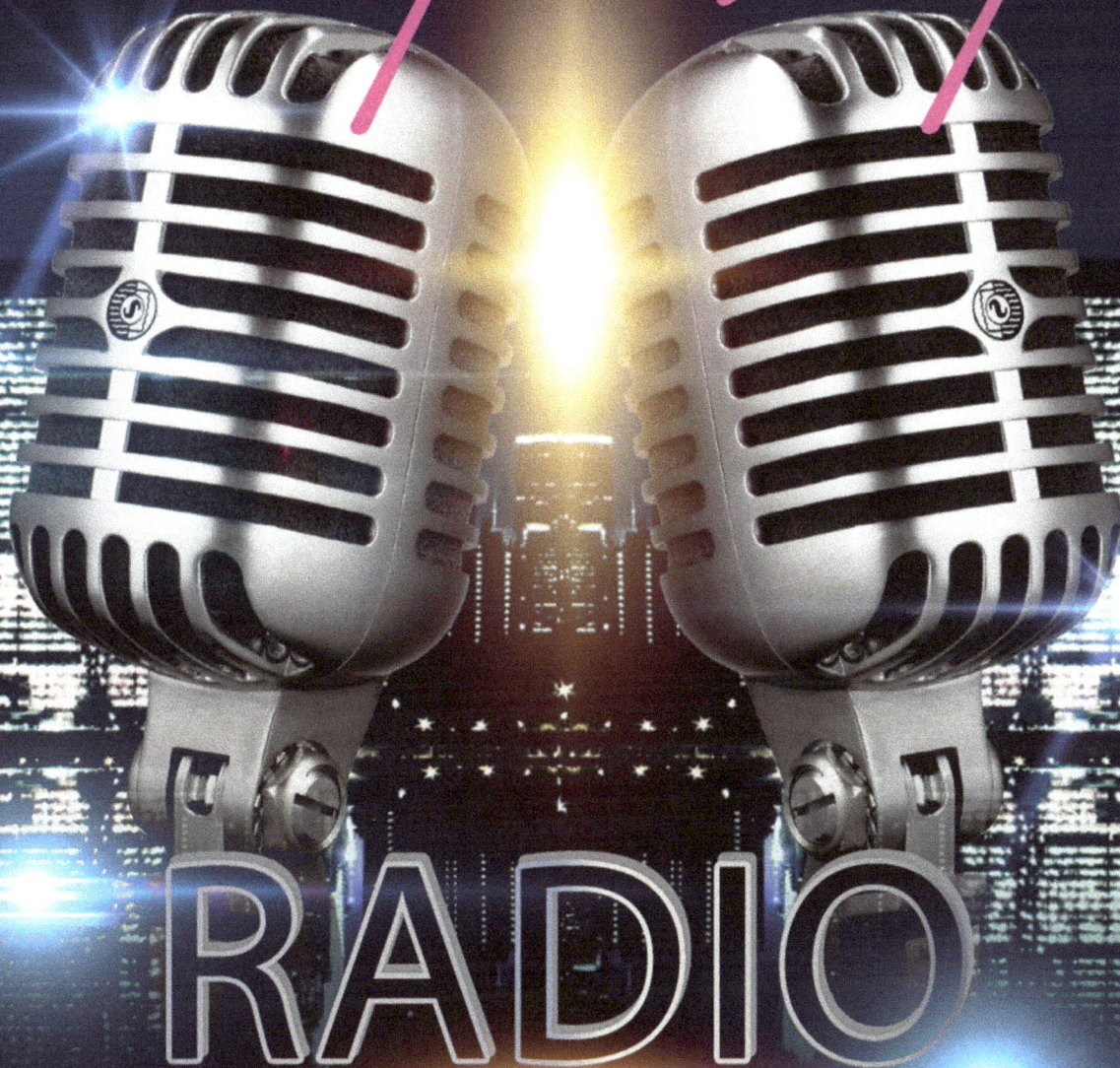

Get the free Pump it up magazine Radio App on your smartphone or tablet, and you'll never miss your favourite music !

POP - ROCK - DANCE - RNB - JAZZ
Available on Google Play Store

www.**PumpItUpMagazine**.com

Pump it up Magazine

TABLE OF CONTENTS

Pump it up

MAGAZINE

PUMP IT UP MAGAZINE —————————

LINKS

WEBSITE
www.pumpitupmagazine.com

FACEBOOK
www.facebook.com/pumpitupmagazine

TWITTER
www.twitter.com/pumpitupmag

SOUNDCLOUD
www.soundcloud.com/pumpitupmagazine

INSTAGRAM
pumpitupmagazine

PINTEREST
www.pinterest.com/pumpitupmagazine

PUMP IT UP MAGAZINE
30721 Russell Ranch Road
Suite 140
Westlake Village,
California 91362
United States
www.pumpitupmagazine.com
info@pumpitupmagazine.com
Tel : (001) (877)841 – 7414 (toll free number)

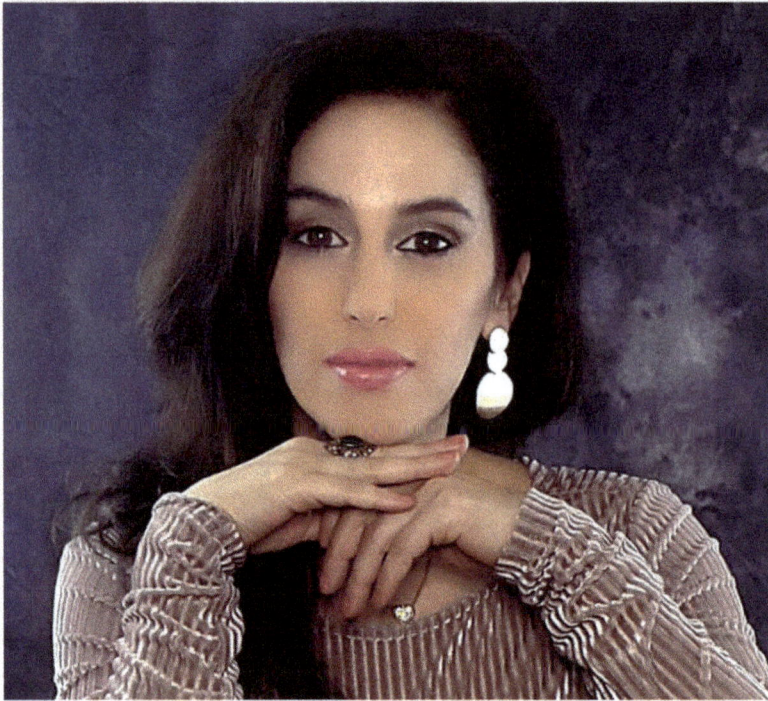

Greetings Pump It Up Magazine Readers,

As I write this editorial we are seeing our nation torn apart by the senseless killing of an African American man. We pray for his family and for all who are suffering from the aftermath of such a tragedy.

Nevertheless I don't want to spend much time on that subject.

Our June and beginning of summer theme is about EDM music and Virtual Reality.

On the cover we have Blazar, an EDM (Electronic Dance Music) Specialist and super talent. His music has been on Billboard charts and had extensive radio airplay.

Also we have an interview with Cori Coppola, producer of the documentary " House of Cardin which is already getting rave reviews. Cori as you can see by her last name comes from a family of historical film makers.

There are more surprises inside, so I won't give it all away, but I invite you to open the pages and browse. I'm sure there is much to pique your interest .

So grab your copy and dig in for a welcome break from all the noise outside and also tune-in to Pump It Up Magazine Radio where we're "playing it proud"!

Be well, safe and blessed!

Best wishes ,

Anissa Boudjaoui

CONTRIBUTORS

FOUNDER & GRAPHIC DESIGNER
Anissa Boudjaoui

EDITOR
Michael B. Sutton
Anissa Boudjaoui

FASHION
Tiffani Sutton

MARKETING
Grace Rose
Corinne Reyes

PARTNERS

Editions L.A.
www.editions-la.com

The Sound Of L.A.
www.thesoundofla.com

Info Music
www.infomusic.fr

Delit Face
www.DelitFace.com

L.A. Unlimited
www.launlimitedinc.com

BLAZAR
Photography by
NICHOLAS ALEXANDER

BLAZAR
"TOMORROW"

*is full of vibrancy and brings positive vibes that fans will surely appreciate.
It is easy to see people putting this song on repeat and adding it to their playlists!!!*

"Tomorrow" starts with beautiful piano lines and is soon coupled with appealing vocals with unique effects applied which help add a great sense of depth. The song flow is consistent and does a great job of transitioning tones from a mellow to an upbeat and energetic nature.

At first the lyrics may appear blurry as you soak in the hypnotizing sonics, but even at some point, the words start to make sense as a catalyst for free association. It's an especially welcome development given electronic music's limitless parameters. BLAZAR's insistence on wringing his grooves for all they're worth keeps the song engaging as a start-to-finish listen in a way that isn't common with today's music. It's worth remembering such a song when you're on a night out partying with your significant other as it taps into that nostalgic magic that makes those moments feel special. "Tomorrow" finds BLAZAR playing across the sound spectrum, with his intense experimentation on a club-ready track providing a fitting impression of his bold personality.

Certainly, a new generation of electronic artists are finding ways to tweak familiar templates, and carve a zig-zag path between respect for their predecessors and a determination to do things their own way. BLAZAR avails himself with resonant chords, one of dance music's most inviting forms and creates something interesting that he explores with emotive piano keys and synthesizers. Intimations of depth also play out in less obvious ways; there is always more here than meets the ear. Needless to say, the more you listen to "Tomorrow" the more fun and enjoyable you find it. The scale of the music is just immense, enough to solidify the everlasting fertility of the style BLAZAR has adopted.

None of it sounds like an exercise in presets, whether musical or emotional, and even though its a lengthy four-minute plus record, BLAZAR makes up for it with rhythmic and melodic texture alongside creativity. There's no saying exactly where. BLAZAR plans to take his music from here but he is focused on giving his audience the ultimate experience. And in order to continue creating interesting and epic sounds that are captivating, he must remain passionate in exploring new musical landscapes with the intention of organically expressing himself as an artist while keeping the listeners entertained.

GREAT TO HAVE YOU ON PUMP IT UP MAGAZINE. PLEASE, INTRODUCE YOURSELF?

Hello, and thank you for having me. I am BLAZAR, I am beaming from Markarian 421.

TELL US ABOUT YOUR NEW ALBUM? AND WHAT'S THE STORY BEHIND IT

This new record is a collaborative effort with some of the coolest behind the scenes producers, engineers, and musicians/artists in music today. I released some music under my name as singer/songwriter "Jerad Finck", and last year I had a single hit the Billboard Charts, charted in 3 formats on Radio, and really just kind of took off on its own. I received a call from Tom Sarig who owns the label AntiFragile Music under Universal/Ingrooves who told me he had heard the song on New Music Friday and offered me a label deal. We discussed my idea for "BLAZAR" which was in my mind in line with Daft Punk. It's more of a collaborative effort that I am helming as both lead Producer/Writer/Artist, but teaming up on every track with all the rad producers, engineers, sessions musicians, artists, mastering engineers, and writers that I've been working with over the last few years as "Jerad Finck" in my solo career.

Only this would be something entirely new, with creative freedom and supported by a label who really was into the idea, and thus BLAZAR was born. I am really into retro synths mixing with modern modulations and just crafting the music beat by beat. The whole idea of the album is this kind of neon burnt out future... a la BladeRunner or Dune and sonically, I wanted it to be a mix of something like The Gorillaz meets Duran Duran meets CHVRCHES meets Michael Jackson, Daft Punk with some of The Knife and Grimes dabbled in there... and maybe sprinkled with some EDM here or there from time to time.

WHAT MAKES YOUR PRODUCTIONS UNIQUE?
AND HOW WOULD YOU DESCRIBE IT?

I think what makes my productions unique is that they are unique. I try to craft every sound. I feel more like an aural chemist, taking sounds from analog synths that I craft as the base of the recipe, and running it through lots of analog gear and saturators, then taking those sounds and creating my own samples from them to modulate with all the modern stuff like Portal, Kontakt, Arcade, Maschine, etc. For me the best part is making every song its own living organism, that has its own fingerprint because for me that is what music is about. The creation of something entirely new that didn't previously exist. I am firmly rooted in Pop, but all of it is very off center Alternative synth wave with some hip hop/funk undertones.
Not really sure what it is, its BLAZAR.

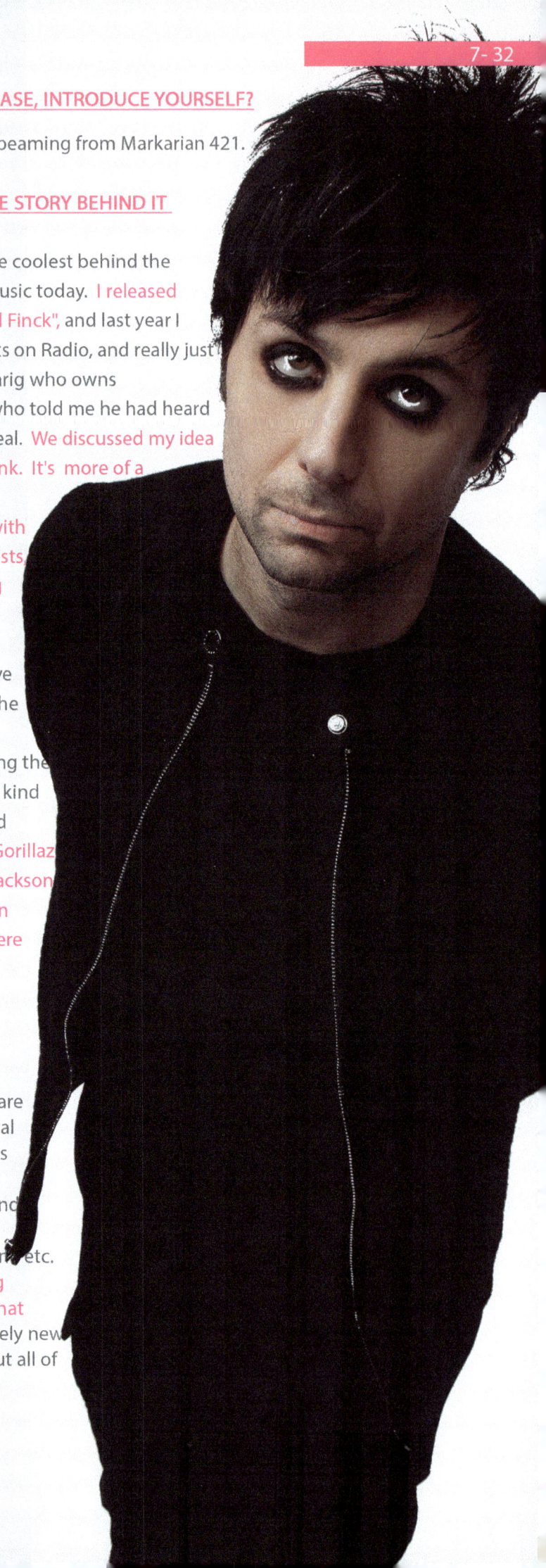

WHO ARE YOUR BIGGEST MUSICAL INFLUENCES? AND ANY PARTICULAR ARTIST/BAND YOU WOULD LIKE TO COLLABORATE WITH IN THE FUTURE?

We love any of the rad producer/artists out there who are really crafting their own sounds and pushing the envelope. We would like to collaborate with The Knife, or Grimes, Daft Punk would be a dream, Billie Eillish, anyone who is living on the edge and pushing it simultaneously.

WHAT DO YOU THINK ABOUT VIRTUAL REALITY?

I think this reality has become a sort of virtual reality with all the insanity going on in the world. It all feels disconnected, without direction, and it just doesn't feel real. The Chaos as we struggle through a pandemic simultaneously with the horrific murder of George Floyd magnified by years of social inequality and foundational/systemic racism coming to a head is something that I don't think we understand the scope of yet. It feels virtual. It's overwhelming.

IF YOU HAD ONE MESSAGE TO GIVE TO YOUR FANS, WHAT WOULD IT BE?

I think the only advice I have to say is to understand that songwriting and artistry in general is work. It is hard work to attempt to be great, and I'm definitely not implying I am, only that talent only carries you a bit of the way. It's that last bit of tenacity that will push you through, and if it's something you want, it takes real work. This comes from simple things like not waiting to be inspired to write, but instead writing every day for the sake of writing better. It's like exercising a muscle.

WHAT'S NEXT FOR YOU? ANY UPCOMING PROJECTS OR LIVE STREAMING?

First of all, just thank you. It was scary as hell to abandon, or put on hold, what I had built as "Jerad Finck" and chase this, but they (AntiFragile) gave me the opportunity and I went for it. The response has been overwhelming. I know it's a new sound for me, but it's where my heart is. I feel like I'm finally putting out the sounds and emotions that I've been trying to convey, and I'm finally able to produce to where I'm not hyper critical, and can start to "listen" to my music again, instead of listening at it. I love that I can collaborate with all of these amazing people, and make this amazing record and have someone helping me to get it out there. So for each and every one of you that has made the jump with me, thank you for continuing on the journey with me.

For all the new fans, thank you for embracing BLAZAR.

To know more about **BLAZAR**, please visit,
WWW.BLAZARMUSIC.COM

And follow BLAZAR on social media
Instagram @iamblazar
Facebook @BlazarOfficial
Spotify Blazar

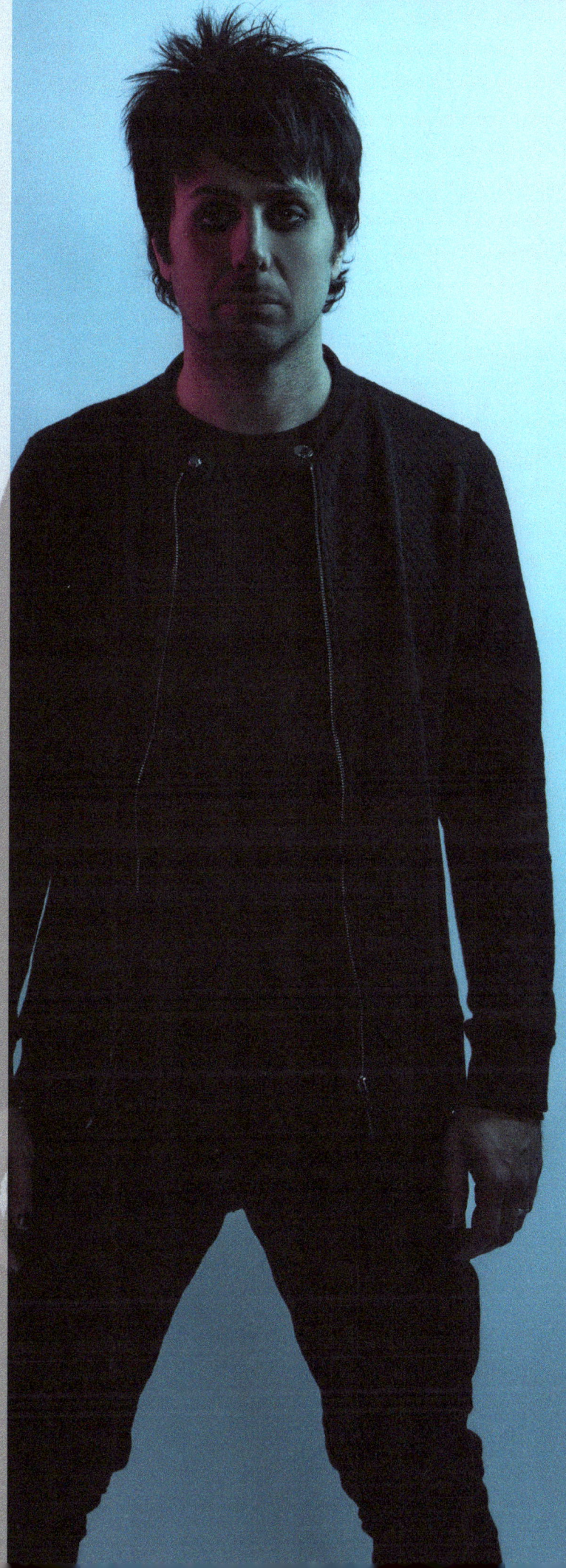

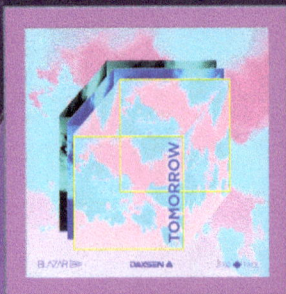

"

TOMORROW by BLAZAR

is full of vibrancy and brings positive vibes that fans will surely appreciate. It is easy to see people putting this song on repeat and adding it to their playlists!!!

Pump it up
Magazine

BLAZAR
"TOMORROW"

OUT NOW!

Spotify · amazon · iTunes

TIDAL

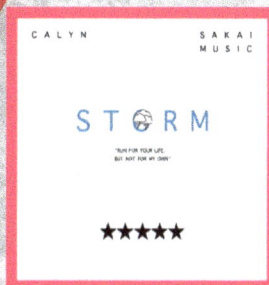

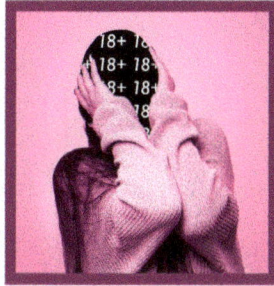

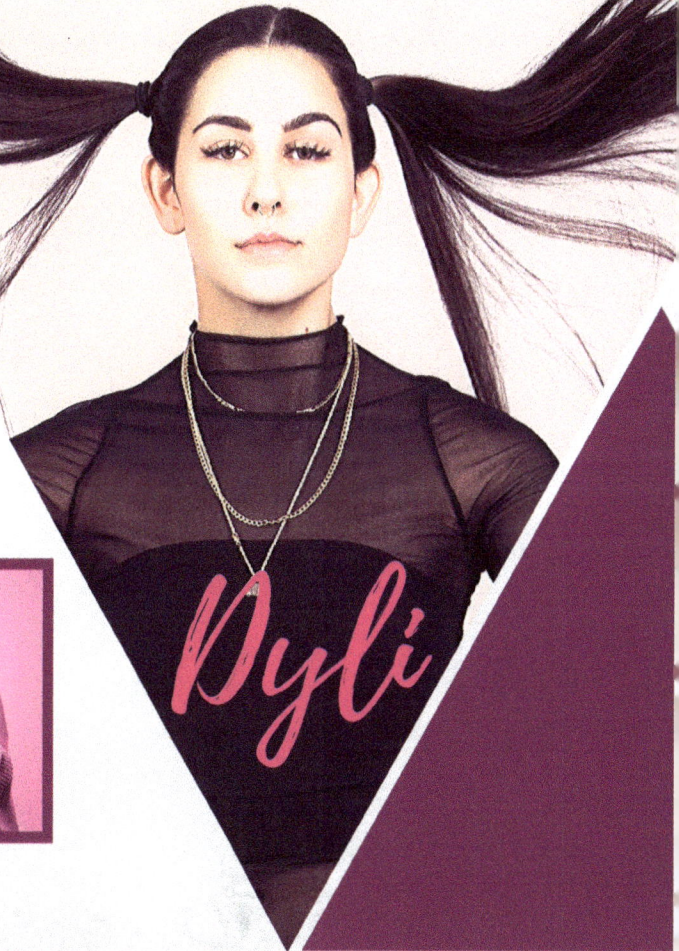

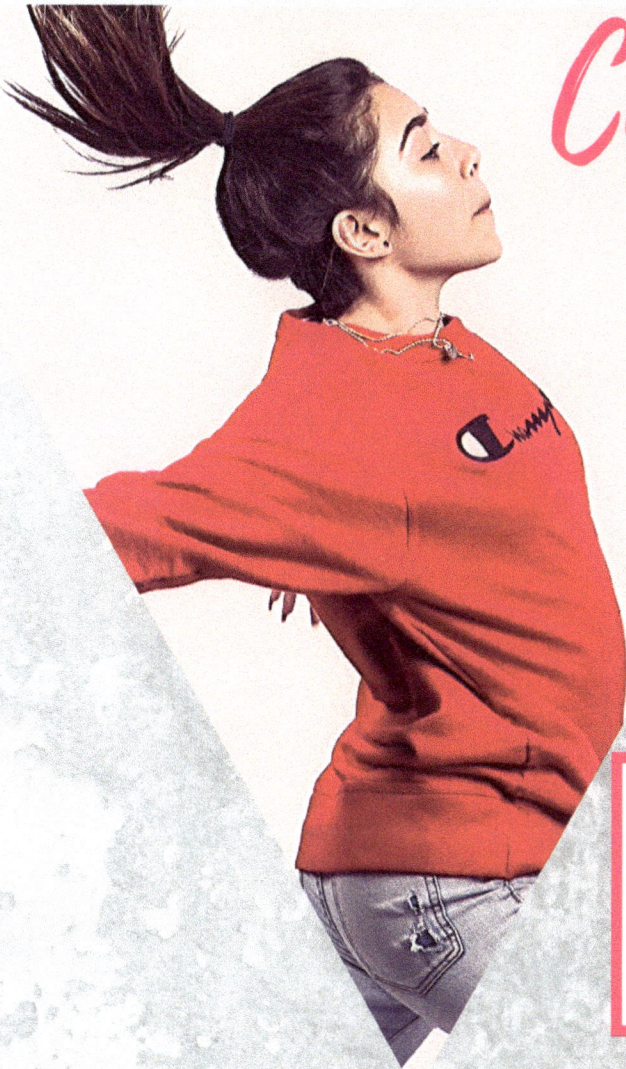

VR & EDM

REVIEW

How virtual reality
is changing the live
music experience

HOW VIRTUAL REALITY IS CHANGING THE LIVE MUSIC EXPERIENCE

Just because your favorite band's live show sold out in minutes, it doesn't mean you have to miss out.

In the last few years, musicians have been able to stream concerts to virtual reality headsets, allowing fans to enjoy the virtual spectacle from the comfort of their homes. Now some VR platforms are going beyond just recreating the live experience, by offering viewpoints and interactions that users could never get if they were at the venue.

Launched in 2018, MelodyVR has built a library of live shows, recorded for streaming to Oculus VR headsets or iPhone and Android devices through its app at a later date. It says it has worked with more than 850 musicians, including Kelly Clarkson, Wiz Khalifa and Lewis Capaldi.

As well as being able to watch from a position in the audience, users can view the concerts as if they were backstage, behind the sound booth, or even on stage with the band. The company has also created more novel experiences; a VR performance by British singer Emeli Sandé displays two images of her simultaneously, one playing the piano and the other singing.

This year, MelodyVR plans to begin offering live streaming via a paid-for virtual ticket, and has designed its own cameras for the task.

"We needed to create [VR cameras] that wouldn't get in the way of the production, but can also survive the variety of elements that could come with a musical performance, whether that is artists jumping around right next to the camera, champagne [being sprayed on them], or fireworks right in front of them," Steven Hancock, co-founder of MelodyVR, told CNN Business.

The company, owned by EVR Holdings, says it holds global VR distribution licenses with major labels Universal Music Group, Sony Music Entertainment and Warner Music Group, as well as Beggars Group.

MelodyVR wouldn't disclose how many users it has, or how many people have watched shows through the platform, but EVR Holdings was valued at around £220 million ($285 million) as recently as January.

It currently operates a pay-per-view model — from $1.99 for one song to around $10 for a whole concert — on Oculus headsets and via its mobile app. This year it will offer a monthly subscription that gives unlimited access to concerts and exclusive sessions. It wouldn't disclose the cost of the subscription.

MelodyVR isn't the only company to deliver VR music performances. Facebook's (FB) Oculus Venues offers live VR experiences of sporting events and comedy shows, and last year, it live streamed a Billie Eilish concert in Madrid. As well as sporting events, NextVR offers "immersive music experiences" filmed in nightclubs and studios. Last year, DJ Marshmello reportedly drew millions of attendees to his virtual show in the online game Fortnite.

A FILM BY BERT MARCUS & CYRUS SAIDI

WHAT WE STARTED

STARRING

MARTIN GARRIX   CARL COX
ERICK MORILLO   MOBY
DAVID GUETTA   AFROJACK
TIESTO   PAUL OAKENFOLD
USHER   ED SHEERAN

EDM DOCUMENTARIES MUST WATCH

These are the best dance music documentaries

I'LL SLEEP WHEN IM DEAD

This Netflix Original Documentary focuses on Steve Aoki and how he grew to where he is today. It was nominated for the 'Best Music Film' at the 2016 Grammy's. It delves into Steve Aoki's upbringing, his family, his friends as well as other associated artists. If you're not a fan of Aoki, this may change your mind.

AFTER THE RAVES

This follows Tommie Sunshine around the world focusing on a different location and DJ's each episode. He goes from Ibiza to Los Angeles, talks with DJ's like Hardwell, Krewella, Dirty South and more, with each episode having a different story. Showing how the rave culture has impacted todays dance music scene.

THIS WAS TOMORROW

This documentary marks the ten year anniversary of the great music festival known as Tomorrowland. Here you learn the impact of music festivals and what electronic dance music means to the people in the business and those that part take in these festivals like Tomorrowland. It follows many individual's experiences, featuring some artists such as Afrojack, David Guetta, Steve Angello, Armin Van Buuren and many more...

ARMIN VAN BUUREN: THIS WAS INTENSE

At the end of the 2013 summer season, Armin van Buuren kicked off a fresh 'Armin Only' world tour, based on his 'Intense' album. 'This Was Intense' follows Armin around the world, showing the ups and downs of being a worldwide touring artist playing sets up to 6 hours long in most cases. If you're a fan of Armin you'll love to see what goes on behind the scenes.

WHaT WE STARTED

A behind the scenes look at Martin Garrix and Carl Cox, focusing on the past three decades. It also includes other individuals such as Erick Morillo, Moby, David Guetta, Steve Angello, Afrojack, Tiesto, as well as pop artists Usher and Ed Sheeran. The film delves into how dance music has integrated with pop culture. It's a good look into the differences and similarities between Carl Cox and Martin Garrix who are arguably on different end of the dance music spectrum.

10 YEARS OF DANCE MUSIC

Toolroom Records is a pioneer in house music today, and they celebrated their 10 year anniversary in 2013 with an enlightening film about their history in EDM, and how America has transformed the foreign sounds into the multi-billion dollar industry it is today. Featuring cameos from some of the biggest names in dance music today, we get a true inside look at the growth of today's scene in this short but sweet documentary.

MUST WATCH

EDM
DOCUMENTARIES

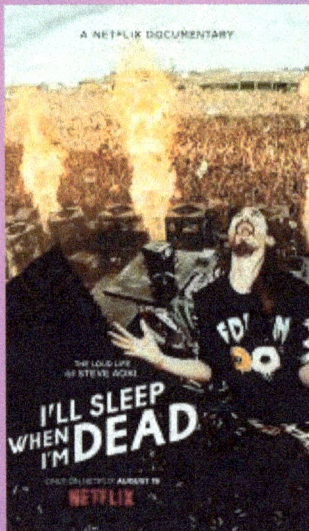

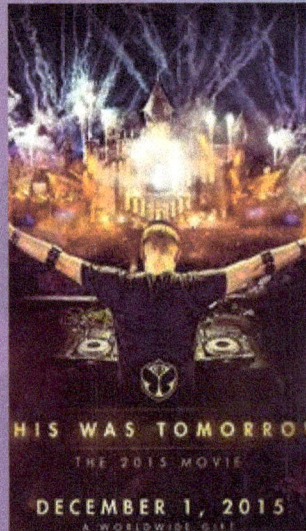

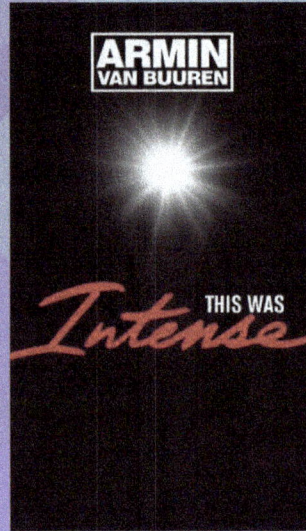

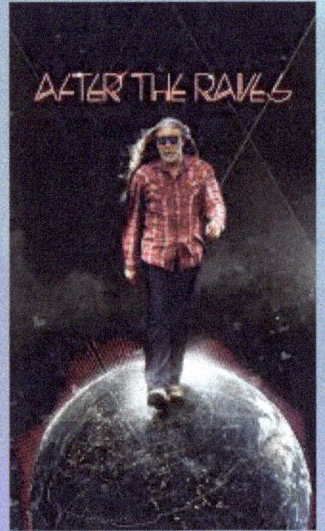

STEVE AOKI | I'LL SLEEP WHEN I'M DEAD
THIS WAS TOMORROW
ARMIN VAN BUREN | THIS WAS INTENSE
AFTER THE RAVES

Pump it up
magazine

*Reach for the stars,
while standing on earth!*

STRATEGIES BEFORE RELEASING YOUR SINGLE

1. CREATE A PLAN

Create at least a three-month marketing plan to promote your new single. Break your plan down into several stages and describe what strategies and tactics you're going to use to promote your single during each stage. Your plan should also contain a timeline and milestones of what you want to accomplish at each stage.

2. PLAN YOUR DEBUT

Are you going to debut your new single by doing a premeire with a music blog or media outlet? Are you going to use radio promotion, social media, record pools, a music video, or a combination of tactics? Decide on how you're going to introduce your new song to the world. Regardless of which method you choose, make sure you leave an impact.

3. DEFINE YOUR NARRATIVE

The narrative of your new single will help you secure press features. Identify your single's unique narrative and tie into your overall brand story. For example, let's say your song is about a woman in a broken relationship who wants to feel loved. The core message of your campaign can be "I Deserve Better." Your narrative would speak of the importance of self-esteem and self-worth in relationships and life.

4. CREATE YOUR VISUALS AND MARKETING MATERIALS

Create your single cover artwork and other marketing materials before the start of your campaign. If you're going to shoot a music video, decide on the concept, filming logistics, release date, and promo plan for your video.

Editions L.A. Design are specialized in all visuals and marketing materials are consistent with your brand. **Contact: anissa@Editions-la.com**

5. REGISTER YOUR WORK

Properly register your single to protect your work, collect your revenue, and track your analytics. Register your song with your performing rights organization, the US Copyright Office, and SoundExchange. You may also want to register your single with Nielsen BDS to track your spins.

6. RADIO PROMOTION

 If you don't have the right contacts, your song has little chance of being played by major radio stations - that is why you need the support of a professional promoter.

Contact info@thesoundofla.com for a successful Radio Campaign

5 Things You Can Do With Merch To Deepen Your Relationship With Your Audience

1. OFFER LIMITED EDITION AND EXCLUSIVE MERCH ITEMS

This is pretty easy to do. If you're touring or have a web store, kick off a new season with items that will only be available for a couple of months or the length of your tour. If you're on tour, create items specific to that tour or album you're promoting — or if you want to get more personal, design a merch item that's indicative of something that's going on in the band's world or represents someone in the band.

2. SPECIALS AT THE MERCH TABLE AT YOUR SHOWS

Buy-one-get-one-half-off - discounts to the first 10 fans (or whatever number makes sense for you) at the merch table - special merch bundles
Deals offered ONLY at the merch table will get your fans coming over for fear of missing out, and it's the perfect time for you or your merch person to have a chat with them if possible. Either way, the fan who's basking in the glow of your awesome show and the deal they're getting may just see something else they want to buy while you have them there.

3. ASK WHAT ITEMS THEY'D LIKE TO SEE ON YOUR NEXT MERCH RUN

Inviting your fans to contribute to ideas will keep them engaged, and also up your chances of selling the merch they suggest. Where should you do this? Wherever you can reach your audience, but we'd recommend email blast and social media.

5. CONTESTS, CALL-TO-ACTION, AND CROWDFUNDINGS

Most of us already do this without realizing it, but creating calls-to-action and contests with merch as the reward is a great way to use merch as a fan engagement tool. Ask fans to share their latest merch purchase on socials and in their network with a special code or link for others to buy it, and if a purchase results because of that share, reward them with more merch, a special item, or a ticket to your next show. Empower your fans with the tool; incentivize them to be your brand ambassadors and they will!

5. CONTESTS, CALL-TO-ACTION, AND CROWDFUNDING

Most of us already do this without realizing it, but creating calls-to-action and contests with merch as the reward is a great way to use merch as a fan engagement tool.
Simply ask fans to post a picture with your merch using a special hashtag, and reward the person with the most likes with a meet-and-greet at your next show.
Empower your fans with the tool; incentivize them to be your brand ambassadors and they will!

YOUR MUSIC CONSULTANT
"YOU BELIEVE, SO DO WE!"

We Can Help You To Grow Your Business

We are a monthly based service, we put faith in artists who has major potential, believed in them, and who are willing to spend their time and own money to work with us in building a successful music career!

Digital Marketing Services

SOCIAL MEDIA - STREAMING SERVICES - MUSIC DISTRIBUTION - PRESS RELEASE - PRESS DISTRIBUTION - PR

Radio Airplay and TV Commercial

TERRESTRIAL AND DIGITAL RADIO CAMPAIGN AL GENRES EXCEPT HEAVY METAL - CABLE TV AND MAJOR NETWORK COMMERCIAL

Licensing & Booking

CONCERTS, LIVE MUSIC, EVENTS, CLUB NIGHTS - RED CARPETS - FOREIGN LICENSING AND SUBOPUBLISHING

Why Choose Us ?

3 DECADES OF MUSIC BUSINESS EXPERIENCE
Platinium and Gold Records

MOTOWN RECORDS
UNIVERSAL
SONY
CAPITOL RECORDS

WE WORKED WITH:
Kanye West - Jay Z - Stevie Wonder - Michael Jackson - Germaine Jackson Smokey Robinson - Dionne Warwick - Cheryl Lynn - The Originals -

📞 **1 -818-514-0038**
(Ext. 1)
Monday - Friday / 9am to 6pm

FIND US :

www.YourMusicConsultant.com
30721 Russell Ranch Road Suite 140 Westlake Village, USA
Email : info@yourmusicconsultant.com

WHY EVERY EMERGING FASHION BRAND
SHOULD HIRE
AN APPAREL LAUNCH CONSULTANCY AGENCY

Let's face it. The world as we know it has drastically changed as we learn to adapt to a new society, compliments of the dreaded menace, the coronavirus.

Every industry has been forced to reinvent itself and restructure. Many apparel businesses have filed for bankruptcy, meeting a rather unfortunate demise. Some are taking advantage to restructure to adjust to the new change. The fashion industry has suffered billions in losses, but there is a silver lining despite all this doom and gloom. There is opportunity and lots of it. *Online business is booming like the great gold rush in California circa 1848.* New brands are in high demand due to many fashion industry veterans closing shop, unable to sustain their overhead. That is where you come in. *The fashion industry needs fresh, hungry, creative talent to reinvent the wheel.*

Your wish to unearth a stellar brand can still be fulfilled. After you have crafted a sellable design to branding perfection, you will need help either selling to the masses or select specialty stores.

Every emerging brand should hire an apparel launch consultancy agency. Why? Apparel brand representation (consultancy) is a necessity to bridge the gap between you and a potential buyer.

Criteria needed:

- Apparel launch consultancy agencies (ALCA) tend to possess coveted buyer contacts with strong relationships.

- ALCAs will perform sales duties much like showrooms but with more personal attention.

- Apparel launch consultancy agencies tend to have less clients or brands to work with hence the personal attention. Showroom representatives tend to represent between 12 to 30 brands with some brands getting ignored.

- Apparel showroom's charge your brand expensive monthly fees to pay to for their contacts, their showroom's rent, monthly parking, on staff reps and other miscellaneous sales tools.

- Apparel brand reps may either charge commission only, a low retainer fee and or a low monthly retainer fee for a confident ROI. Trade show participation fees can be extra depending on the size of your collection and materials needed.

Independent apparel brand representatives such as L.A. Unlimited & Associates offer consultative services at no extra cost. WWW.LAUNLIMITEDINC.COM

Before you embark on launching your brand, you will need to hire an apparel consultancy agency to work with apparel and or accessory buyers, walk you through the sales process, interpret industry sales terms and bring your brand revenue. Its highly recommended to research what type of apparel launch consultancy agency would be best for your brand. Industry specific search engines like Find Fashion Rep (www.findfashionrep.com) and We Connect Fashion (www.weconnectfahion.com) are databases that lists apparel consultants and sales representatives with specific criteria.
THE TIME IS NOW!

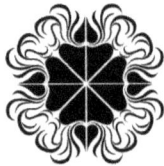

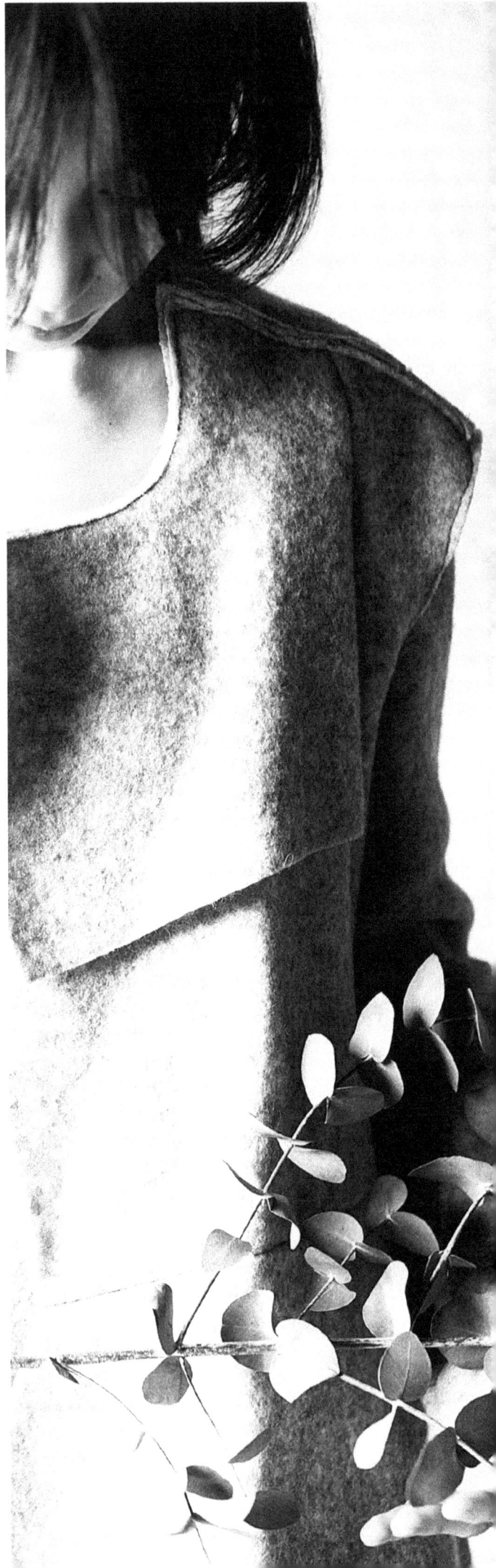

LET'S GET IN SHAPE!

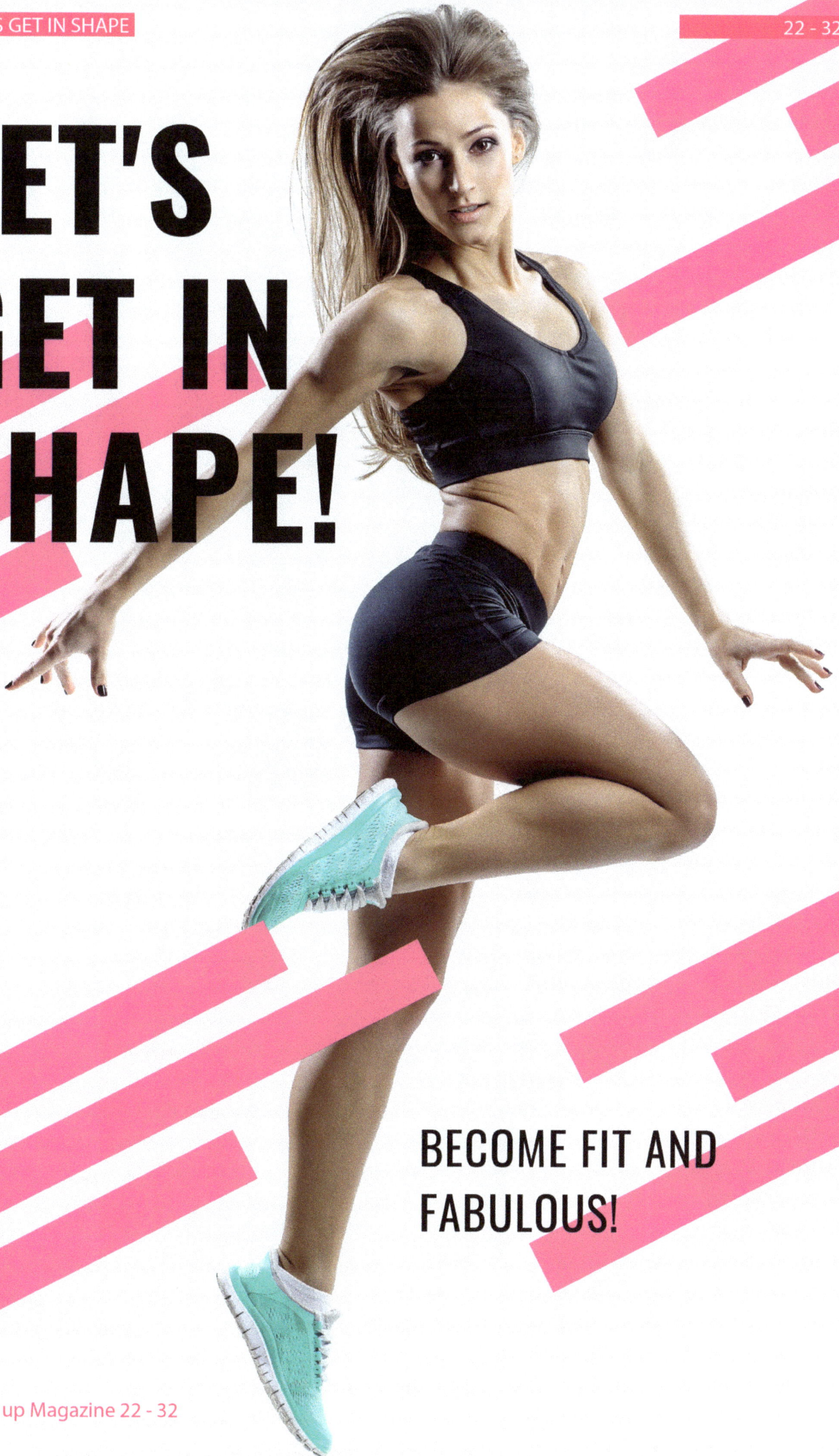

BECOME FIT AND FABULOUS!

Abs-olutely
Amazing Core
Exercises
for a Flat Stomach

Take a break from countless crunches. Getting a strong, sleek midsection takes the right mix of ab workouts for women that work together to tone the entire area!

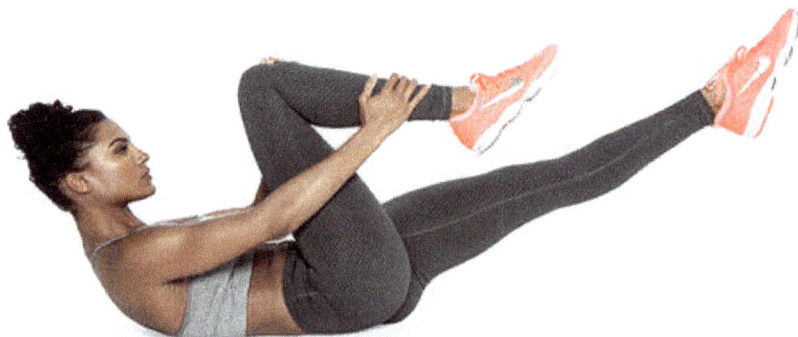

Sets: 2 to 3 Reps: 8 to 10

Lie faceup on floor with arms by sides.
Curl head and shoulders off floor, then raise extended arms and legs at a 45-degree angle to start.
Keeping upper body lifted throughout, bring right knee toward chest and reach right hand outside of right ankle and left hand inside of right knee.
Switch sides and repeat to complete 1 rep.

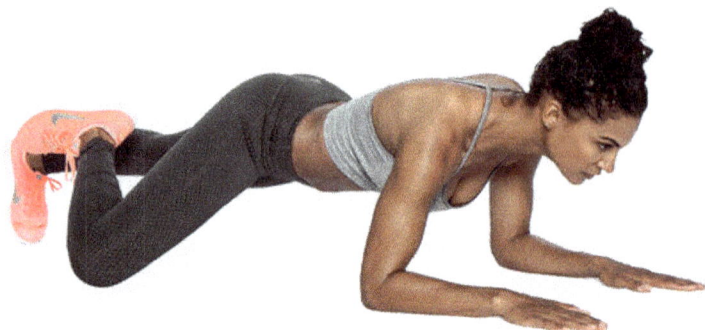

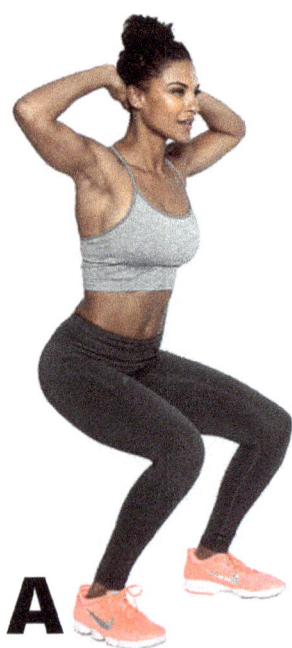

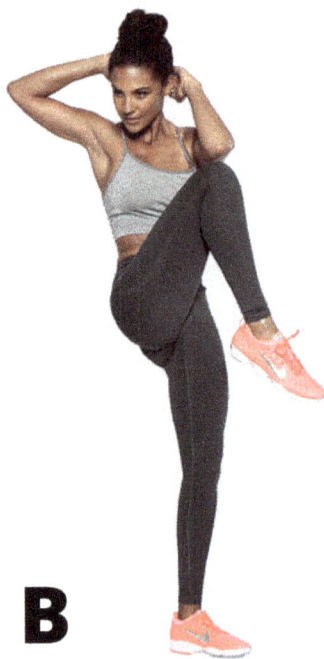

Sets:2 to 3 Reps:8 to 10

Start on floor in forearm plank position, body balancing on forearms and toes, palms flat.
Keep hips level and bend right knee out to side toward right triceps.
Return to plank.
Switch sides and repeat to complete 1 rep.

Sets:2 to 3 Reps: 12

Stand with feet hip-width apart, elbows bent out to sides and fingertips behind ears.

B.Squat slightly (bend knees about 45 degrees, and avoiding these 6 common squat mistakes) to start, then shift weight to left leg as you stand, lifting bent right knee and rotating torso toward right so left elbow and right knee meet in front of chest.
Return to start position, switch sides, and repeat to complete 1 rep.

A

B

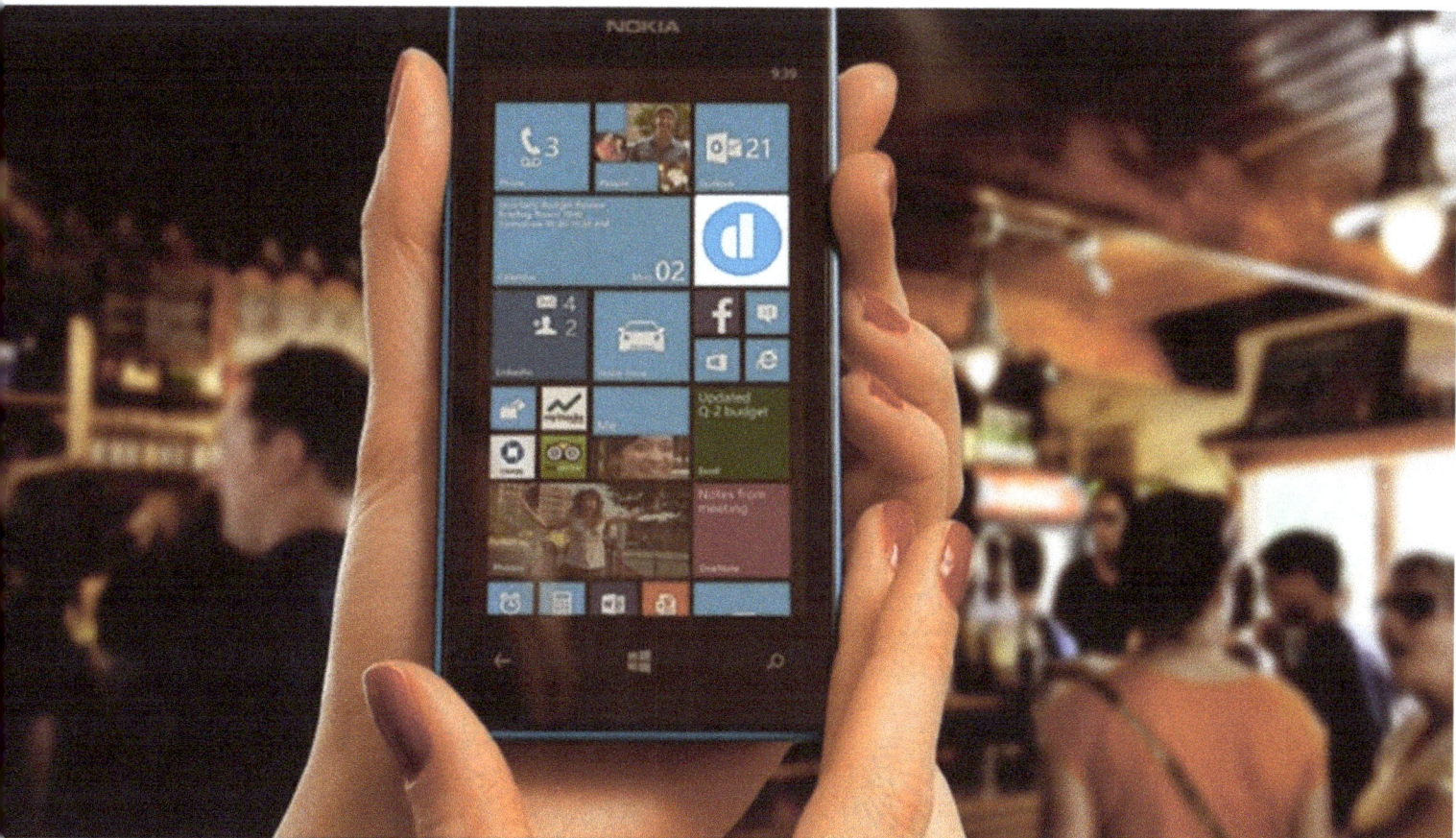

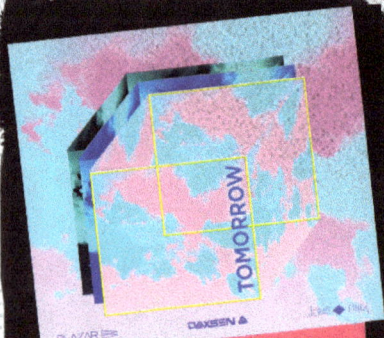

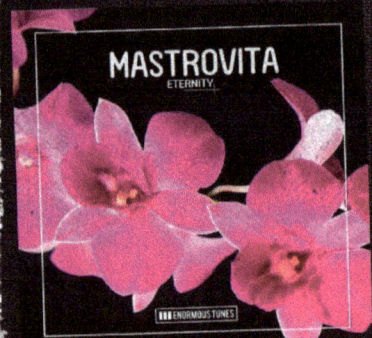

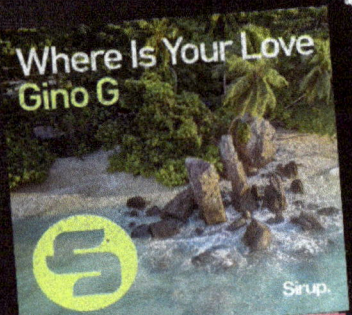

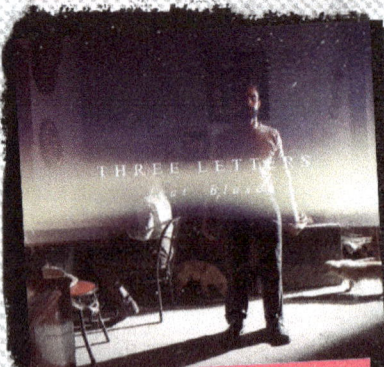

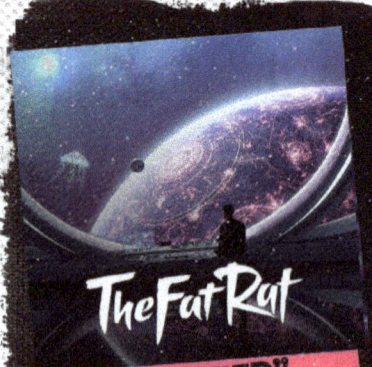

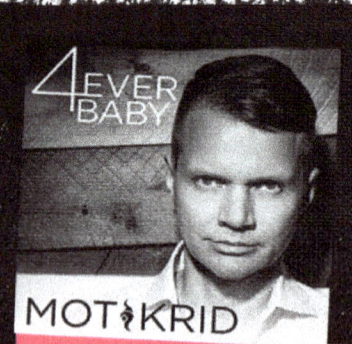

IN STORES NOW

RANDY HALL
A New Way Of Love
REMIX

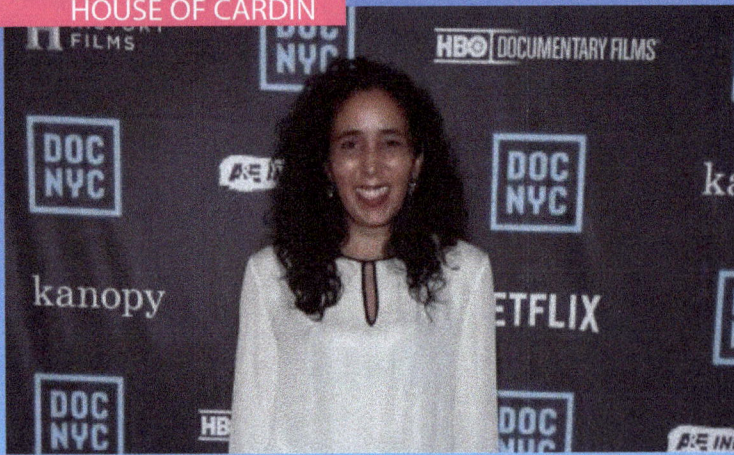

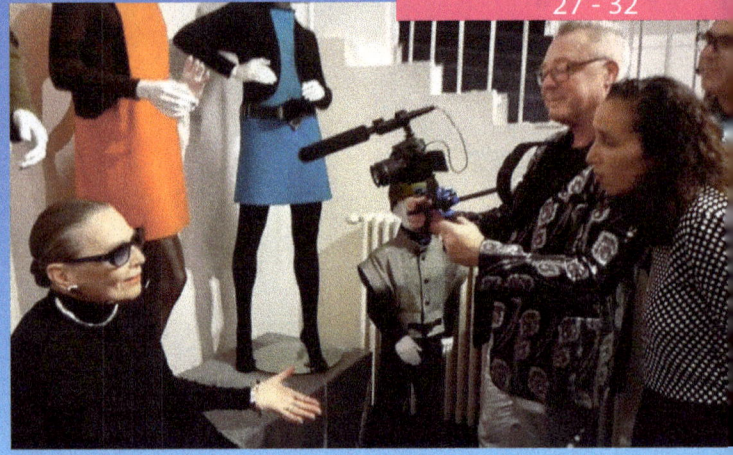

Interview With

Cori Coppola

Writer & Producer in Paris / Producer for the documentary "House of Cardin"
on the life and work of fashion designer Pierre Cardin.

Pierre Cardin

WHY DID YOU DECIDE TO BE A PRODUCER ABOVE ALL OTHER INDUSTRY JOB ROLES?

Being a Producer wasn't really something I chose to do. I think to some extent, it chose me. I started out in the visual effects industry as a production assistant, and I worked my way up the ladder to production coordinator and eventually ended up as a full producer. In the US, I primarily worked on large-scale productions, and when I moved to France, initially I worked for an international film and television sales market for Central and Eastern Europe. We branched out into China and Russia as well, but eventually I did go back to visual effects, this time on the commercial and advertising end.

DID YOU ATTEND FILM SCHOOL OR STUDY FILM AT UNIVERSITY?

No, interestingly enough, I have been reading The Outliers by Malcolm Gladwell, and he discusses how many people become experts in their line of work if they devote at least 10,000 hours. My stepfather growing up was a film and television director and producer, and my mother worked as a producer as well. I spent time nearly every week after school on a set somewhere, and for a while, my mother had an office on the Zoetrope lot where I would run around watching shoots, hanging out in the editing rooms and just basically observing; so I think I absorbed a certain amount of production know-how which to my mind is the best way to really learn something from the inside out. Producing is something I really just enjoy doing, and I probably have something close to 10,000 of production time behind me even if some of that time was just hanging out on sets as a child.

WHAT WAS YOUR FIRST JOB IN FILM AND HOW DID YOU PROGRESS TO PRODUCER?

My very first job in film was working for Jeff Kleiser and Diana Walczak in visual effects. I literally started out answering the phone, copying scripts, making coffee and running various errands for the office. We were working in the Berkshires on a project with Doug Trumbull, and then later, I worked for them out of their office in Los Angeles where we worked on a ton of high-profile projects. I was a production assistant and coordinator and got to meet some amazing directors, watching dailies, taking notes, etc. It wasn't until years later when I was in Paris working at BUF that I became an in-house producer, and then later I went over to Partizan. These were wonderful learning experiences, but I put my career on hold for several years after having children.

WHAT DO YOU LOOK FOR IN A SCRIPT?

For the moment, I am mostly looking at documentary stories to tell, so I look for things that I can be passionate about, not just from a story-telling point of view but also topics that I think will be fun to research and share.

CAN YOU TELL US ABOUT YOUR LATEST DOCUMENTARY " HOUSE OF CARDIN"?

House of Cardin is probably my favorite project that I have ever worked on. There are some projects that come together as if by magic, and the directors P. David Ebersole and Todd Hughes are themselves magical people who bring a lot of excitement and joy to everything they do. I also enjoyed getting to do many of the French-language interviews.

The people that we interviewed included names like Sharon Stone, Naomi Campbell, Philipe Starck and Jean-Paul Gaultier. It was the kind of project that made me just jump out of bed in the morning excited for the day ahead. I am really proud of the final product and am excited for it to come out, if not in theaters, then virtually.

HOW DO YOU SELECT A DIRECTOR?

I look for someone who has a distinct vision because that is what really carries a project forward. There has to be passion because that trickles down to the rest of the crew. I do think that is a natural quality that directors have which is a guiding force in what projects they themselves are drawn to.

OBVIOUSLY FROM THE SOUND OF YOUR LAST NAME YOU ARE RELATED TO FRANCIS FORD COPPOLA. HAVE YOU OR DID YOU EVER SEEK HIS ADVICE IN FILM PRODUCTION OR DIRECTION?

No, I have never really asked him about anything related to making films. By pure chance, it was my family though that bought the film for North American distribution. It was funny to get in to the meeting and hear my cousin Robert Schwartzman saying hello so unexpectedly. I had not thought to tell anyone in the family that I was working on the film, so I felt like it was a natural fit for our movie to be distributed by one of my cousins.

WHAT ADVICE WOULD YOU GIVE TO THOSE HOPING TO PURSUE A CAREER IN PRODUCING?

think that anyone who wants to work in the film industry or any industry for that matter should be totally in love with what they are doing because it is not a job for the faint of heart.

It demands a lot of persistence, belief in your project which can literally take years to get made, and you need be motivated by the vision of the director.

You can't get out of bed for a paycheck. You should be doing something that matters to you so much that you'd do it no matter what because at the end of the day, you want to be happy with your choices about the projects you are working on.

Life is short – you don't have time for regrets!

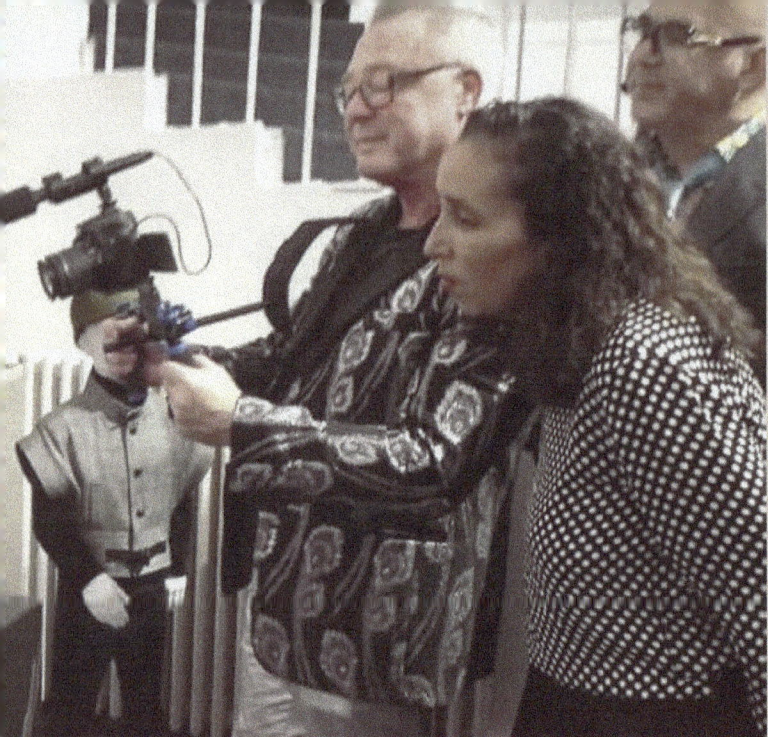

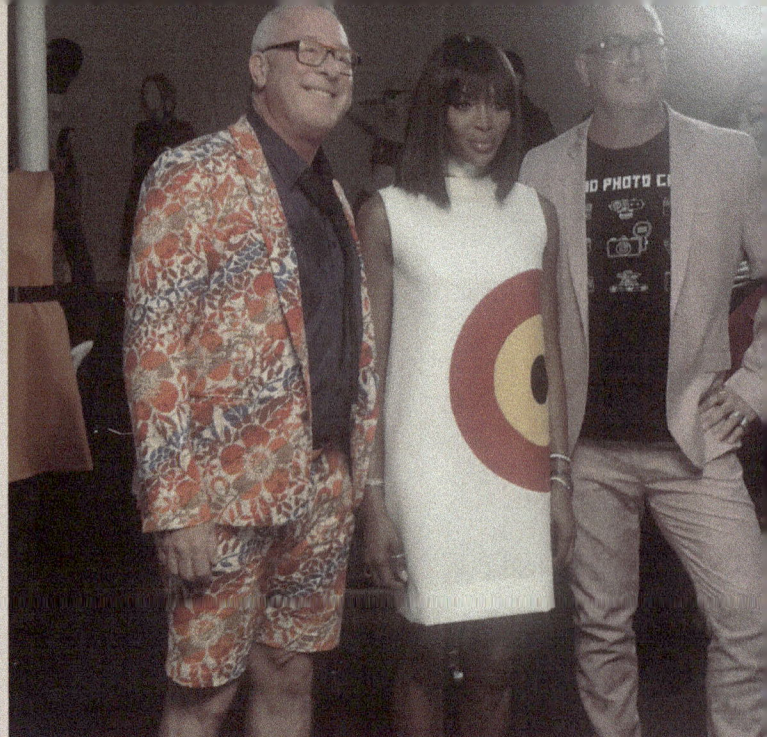

HOUSE OF CARDIN

PRODUCED BY CORI COPPOLA

House of Cardin is a globetrotting journey across the decades, examining the modernist styles he pioneered. Featuring Pierre Cardin, Naomi Campbell, Amy Fine Collins, Alice Cooper, Jean-Paul Gaultier, Jean-Michel Jarre, Yumi Katsura, Hanae Mori, Guo Pei, Jenny Shimizu, Phillippe Starck, Sharon Stone, Kenzo Takada, Trina Turk, Dionne Warwick.
Directed by P. David Ebersole, Todd Hughes.

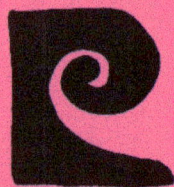

@HOUSEOFCARDIN

Pierre Cardin

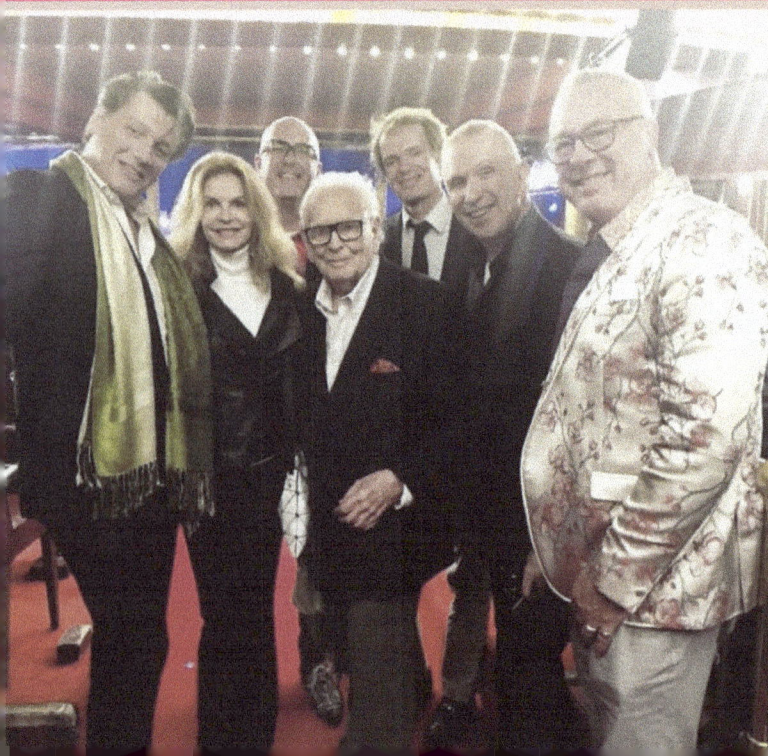

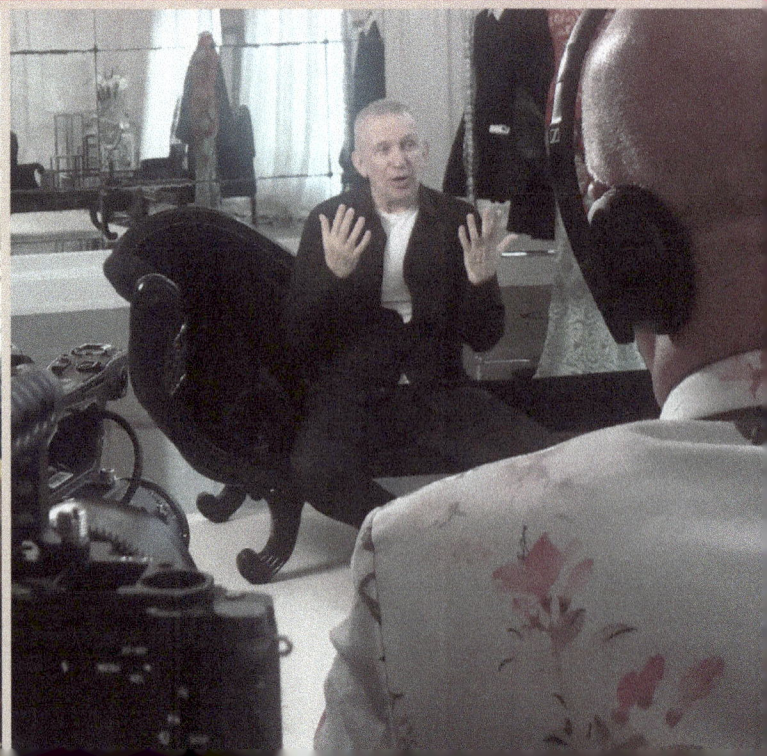

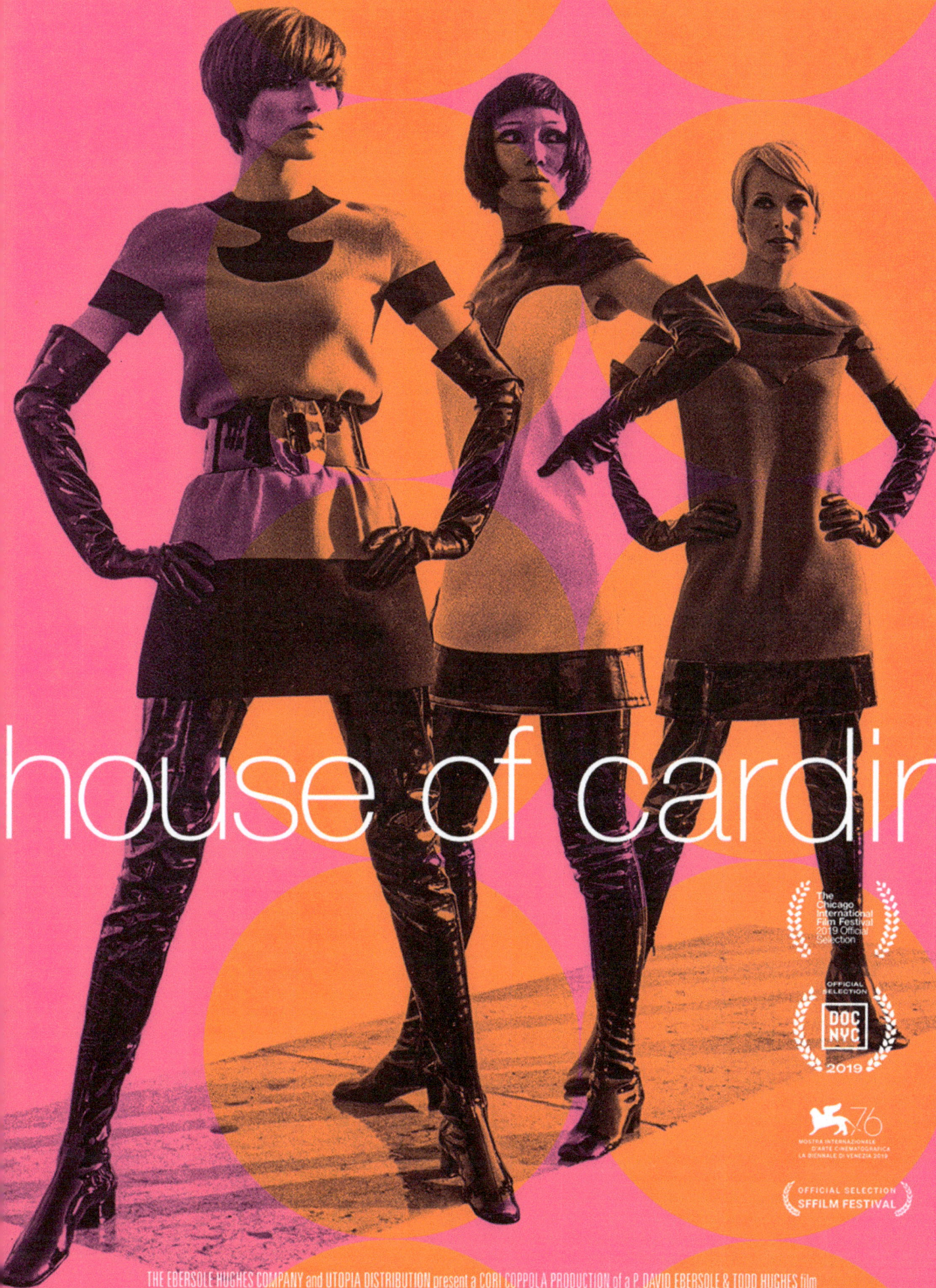

THOUGHTS ON
GEORGE FLOYD PROTESTS

Will we one day wake up to realize that perhaps " we" are the change we're looking for? Do we really know the answer? is there really a solution? What the hell does the voice of truth really sound like? Look like? Do we really know?

Preachers, teachers, politicians do you really know the answer? Are you praying to have chairs rearranged on the Titanic? Are we really that surprised that people are angry and full of rage? Did you see that disturbing video?

While many of us cried and became full of shock at the sight of Mr. Floyd (yes I said Mr. Floyd) gasping for his every breath, until his last! Did you look into the eyes of the perpetrator? Did you see the look in his eyes? This monster has his hand in his pocket, knee on Floyd's neck with all of his weight into it, and looking straight ahead at bystanders as if he had just "won" a WWE match. Mission accomplished! Black man down! Victory!

And as if to say, " now what you gonna do about it? Something more than, " it just ain't right" is going on. This looks premeditated, an expected outcome! Then an unidentified man dressed in black starts breaking windows with a hammer and telling people there is free stuff inside and then walks away into the distance? Then a peaceful protest turns into a riot? Wake Up! And smell the coffee, cappuccino, tea, or hot chocolate or whatever! But destroying private property is where u draw the line. It ain't right, but I understand. I think I do but don't agree or condone it.

We talk about " prayer" as the answer to racism and violence and seeking God's answer? Or a quote from MLK or whomever, Well how many times in the Bible do we read of God's answer with telling one tribe to strike down another tribe. Jesus saying I came not to bring peace, but a sword. But also saying " Blessed are the peacemakers". How many religions have taken the term God's " chosen people" to further their agenda of racism? Or violence?

In all of these Scriptural passages, God supposedly makes violent moves when one of two things happens: either His (God's)honor has been offended, or a nation's or race's well-being is at stake. How are we to read into this?

Maybe they are not really commandments from " God" but our human projections on him. So if literally taken as the word of " God" This would justify one race', or nation or religion to believe that they are God's " Chosen".

I'm not convinced that we can solve the problems of today with yesterday's solutions or the same old answers. New questions may be in order. For instan

Who is God? Who am I ? Where do I fit in this seemingly scripted life? How did we get to all this? Is this it? Is this the best we can do? Is there other information for us to tap into other than CNN, Fox News, MSNBC, and others and Social Media?

Where do I go from here? How can I help myself or another feel better, love better, be better.. what the heck is " better"?

STEVIE WONDER SAID IT BEST.
"TEACHERS KEEP ON TEACHING, PREACHERS KEEP ON PREACHING, WORLDS KEEP ON TURNING TILL WE REACH THE HIGHEST GROUND! " WHEREVER OR WHATEVER THAT IS!

www.ingramcontent.com/pod-product-compliance
Lightning Source LLC
Chambersburg PA
CBHW040802050426
42336CB00066B/3451